Bella Vida

A Beautiful Life with
Homeopathic HGH Therapy

By Dr. Howard Peiper

Editor: Nina Anderson, SPN

Printed in the United States of America

Published by Safe Goods
561 Shunpike Rd.
Sheffield, MA 01257
888 217-7233

Bella Vida *A Beautiful Life with Homeopathic HGH Therapy* is not
intended as medical advice. No claims are made for the ability of
Homeopathic HGH to treat, cure or prevent any disease. No promise
is made for health, and no diagnostic or health claims are stated.
This literature is for informational purposes only and is not meant to
diagnose, or prescribe for, any health condition. Cease taking HGH
or any product, and consult a health care practitioner if there is a
consistent, negative change of symptoms. Always see a health care
professional for matters relating to your health. The FDA has not
evaluated this information.

Table of Contents

I have been keenly interested in preserving and restoring the body to health and have made it the main focus of my medical life. I scrutinize each and every "miracle treatment" that comes along, and was pleasantly surprised at the amount of research behind the beneficial effects of homeopathic human growth hormone. As a firm believer in utilizing a more natural approach to healing, I find the benefits of the homeopathic HGH therapy in persons 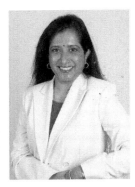 concerned with the effects of aging, to be realized as indicated with virtually no side effects. As a medical professional, this allows me to speak about the supplement with confidence.

Dr. Peiper has outlined the benefits of this remarkable anti-aging method in a comprehensive manner, and has expanded its scope by listing potential ingredients that may be utilized to potentize HGH's efficacy. His treatment of a suggested protocol for a healthy lifestyle was in line with current natural dietary guidelines. For example, I have been advocating pH balance as a key to homeostasis in the body and was very impressed that he included this subject matter. Bella Vida is extremely up-to-date and the inclusion of The Boulder Study and others lays the foundation for any practitioner to have faith that the product will produce the desired results.

As our aging population grows exponentially, every practitioner should read this book and consider putting it in a key position on their reference bookshelves. Individuals as well, should use this book as a tool for self-education in the realm of what to do to help the body avoid the degenerative pitfalls of aging.

Thank you Dr. Peiper for providing us with this potentially life-changing information.

-Dr. Vijaya Nair, M.D., FAMS, M.S. (Epid) Author of *Prevent Cancer, Strokes, Heart Attacks and Other Deadly Killers.*

CHAPTER ONE

THE KEY TO A BEAUTIFUL LIFE

Do you fear declining health and the onset of wrinkles and other telltale signs of aging? Most of us would love to feel and look young forever. Since that is not reality, let us explore the facts behind aging and look at ways to turn back the clock.

We know about the destructive effects of free radicals on our cells, and the importance of antioxidants in neutralizing this damage. In addition, the decline of hormone production that begins in our mid-thirties, plays a significant factor in the way we age.

Many studies have shown a direct correlation between aging and a lack of Growth Hormone (GH). Our body reaches a maximum production of GH during puberty. As we enter our 30's, we notice several changes in the body due to a diminished GH. People may gain weight and have a harder time getting rid of it than before. Your body also weakens and you are more prone to injury than you were when you were young. From 40 on, your body starts showing all the signs of aging, as this hormone lessens even more. Our waist gets fatter and wrinkles become more prevalent. Our Growth Hormone is still being produced, but not released while the production of others is in decline. The challenge is to restore our youthful levels of GH which has been kept in a sequestered state.

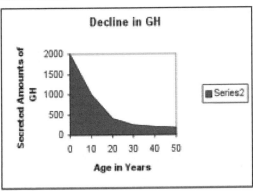

Results that could be achieved by restoring active levels of GH include:

- Reducing wrinkles
- Restoring lost hair and nail color
- Improving vision
- Elevating mood and improving sleep
- Normalizing blood pressure
- Assist in wound healing
- Restoring the size of liver, pancreas, heart and other organs that shrink with age
- Increased life expectancy
- Enhancing sexual performance
- Improving exercise capacity
- Improving quality of deep sleep
- Enhancing energy levels
- Tighter, more hydrated, smoother skin
- Decrease in body fat
- Increase in lean body mass
- Strengthened immune system
- Sharper memory and concentration
- Improving cholesterol profile
- Reducing appetite
- Enhanced feeling of well being
- Reduced cellulite

CHAPTER TWO

WHAT IS HUMAN GROWTH HORMONE?

H GH (Human Growth Hormone) is a naturally occurring substance in the body which is secreted by the pituitary gland. As we get older, production gradually slows over time. GH affects almost every tissue in the body. Pituitary tumors, chronic illness, side effects of therapy for other medical conditions, and processes associated with aging all can contribute to reduced pituitary function and decreased production of growth hormone. GH is the "master hormone" controlling many organs and body functions and is directly responsible for stimulating tissue repair, cell replacement, brain functions, and enzyme function. Symptoms of Growth Hormone deficiency include fatigue, decreased lean body mass, abdominal obesity and weight gain, decreased physical strength, decreased muscle mass, reduced cardiac performance, impaired sense of wellbeing, and poor sleep.[1]

In 1912 Dr. Harvey Cushing discovered Growth Hormone but it wasn't used therapeutically until the 1960s when Dr. Maurice Raben gave GH to a child who was growth deficient. The boy began growing normally. Dr. Raben then gave GH to a 35 year old who experienced new vigor, and sense of wellness. The drawback to administering this on a large scale was acquiring a supply. The only source for the hormone was to extract it from the pituitary gland of human cadavers. Each gland only contributed a few drops and so to obtain enough for just a single injection was very time consuming, and also very expensive.

In 1985, biosynthetic human growth hormone replaced pituitary-derived human growth hormone for therapeutic use in the U.S. and elsewhere. After thirty years of experience with both children and adults deficient in Growth Hormone, no significant side effects had been experienced, and so researchers began giving GH to healthy adults. The New England Journal of Medicine published a study by Dr. Daniel Rudman at the Medical College of Wisconsin in Milwaukee. He had patients in the age bracket of 61 to 81 in his study. These men, without any exercise, lost an average of 14% body fat, gained 8.8% lean muscle, regained lost bone mass, thickened their skin by 7%, lost wrinkles, and re-grew failing liver tissue by 19%. In summary growth hormone returned flabby, frail old men to their younger, healthier, sleeker selves. It was estimated that this 6-month therapy reversed twenty years of aging.

In the controlled group, some individuals did not receive any injections, these individuals aged normally. The exact published quote in the New England Journal of Medicine – "The effects of six months of human growth hormone on lean body mass and adipose-tissue were equivalent in magnitude to the changes incurred during 10-20 years of aging".

The drawback for this therapy was the price of the injections. At $15,000 to $30,000 a year only the wealthy could afford it. Then in 1998 came another tremendous breakthrough; researchers were able to create an oral form. And they came with a list of potential hazards: allergic response, massive bleeding, edema or swelling, blood sugar problems (either too high or too low), gastrointestinal problems, cancer, heart problems, extremely low blood pressure to name a few.

Medical science alludes to Growth Hormone as the master hormone. Hormones are chemical messengers, traveling through the blood stream and involved in all aspects of the body's activity - metabolism, growth, mood and sexual function to name a few. They also help to maintain health, regulate the vital organs, and promote healing and repair. Being the master hormone, GH affects virtually all areas of the body — influencing the growth of cells, bones, muscles and organs.

Growth hormone is a 191-amino acid, single-chain polypeptide that is synthesized, stored, and secreted by somatotropic cells within the lateral wings of the anterior pituitary gland. Somatotropin (STH) refers to the growth hormone produced naturally in animals, whereas the term somatropin refers to growth hormone produced by recombinant DNA technology, and is abbreviated "HGH" in humans.[2]

4

GH is a protein that consists of amino acids identified as the peptide hormones, which differ from other proteins, as most of them are made up of lesser proteins which are linked together. This protein, however, is created as one extended chain and may consist of some two hundred amino acids. Effects of growth hormone on the tissues of the body can generally be described as anabolic (building up). Like most other protein hormones, GH acts by interacting with a specific receptor on the surface of cells. Bio-engineered HGH starts with a natural plasmid purified culture (can be non-animal) that is formed, and the bioengineered DNA for Growth Hormone is inserted where it "infuses" in the culture. Over time, it develops the 191 single chain amino acid patterns that duplicate human Growth Hormone. The inert powder is removed and the rest (HGH) is freeze-dried and later solubilized for injection (or for homeopathic or oral molecular use.) This made it possible for GH to be more readily available.

There are over 28,000 written studies reporting many positive results on human Growth Hormone. However, GH came with side effects. Dr. Edmund Chein devised a low dose (LD), high frequency (HF) system of GH therapy and by giving his patients a very low dose, once in the morning and once prior to sleep, six days a week, the GH did not produce side effects. From 1994 to 1996, Dr. Chein collaborated with Dr. Leon Cass Terry and carried out studies of 800 patients using this low dose, high frequency approach with extremely positive results. This research was leading towards homeopathic applications.

CHAPTER THREE

WHY HOMEOPATHIC HGH?

In the early 1800s Samuel Hahnemann, M.D. developed homeopathy. Homeopathy is recognized as a safe, effective way to help the body, and is also the second most prominent form of medicine in the world. This form of treatment encourages the body to clear itself. In contrast, allopathic medicine artificially suppresses symptoms of disease and is sometimes toxic to the body.

The word "homeopathy" means, "like treats like." A symptom that results from taking a substance in its raw form can be alleviated by taking that same substance in a highly diluted and properly succussed form. This is similar to how vaccinations work. Small is better: the body itself breaks food down to microscopic amounts in order to transport nourishment to minute cells. If we use the example of a thyroid hormone that can be as small as 50 to 100 millionths of a gram in size. Despite the small size, bodily metabolism is maintained.

There is no toxicity associated with homeopathics since they use minute amounts of a substance and encourage the body to bring itself into balance. Years of research have shown that homeopathic remedies work similarly to allopathic counterparts but without the side effects. They have been used successfully to treat various physical and emotional problems and are also very effective when used topically. In clinical practice, homeopathic drugs have demonstrated effectiveness repeatedly, bringing the body closer to homeostasis.[3]

Homeopathic potency is important. It is a dilution process where you are basically getting an extremely small dose of a substance that the body reacts to without side effects. The decimal potency is denoted by an X. You begin with a base (ex: purified water, alcohol, glycerin, lactose or sucrose) and add two or more with the Growth Hormone. Then you succuss (shake) the mixture up to 100 times. This creates a 1X potency. Take another 1 part of this potency and combine with 9 parts of the base, succuss it another 100 times and you get a 2X potency. If you see a C potency on a homeopathic remedy, this means that the dilution is 1 to 99 and is more potent.

Hormesis is the term scientists use to describe small doses of substances that create a beneficial response. According to the Arndt Schultz Law, substances vary in action depending on whether the concentration is high, medium, or low. High concentrations inhibit; medium concentrations suppress; and low, or minute, concentrations stimulate. Homeopathic substances work naturally and gently in the body. But be diligent in choosing a product because some may have an "X" or a "C" after a number to show that a substance has been diluted, but it may not be a homeopathic, because it has not been properly succussed.

When GH is combined with an oral homeopathic preparation, researchers discover better results without any side effects. Many people who have taken homeopathic GH have reported similar results to those taking injectable forms of GH. Because of the high dilutions the homeopathic potencies of GH may become even more effective in the body since scar tissue may not interfere with its absorption. Factors that contribute to tissue and organ scarring include a lack of nutrients, diseases, nitrites, smoking, excessive alcohol intake, surgery, old internal wounds and high LDL cholesterol levels. I suspect that this is a reason why GH is not produced at acceptable levels in people with these types of scaring.

During the homeopathic process the energies and properties of the HGH molecules are transferred into the molecules of the base solution. The solution becomes potentiated by the human growth hormone and possesses the properties and abilities of the HGH. This homeopathic solution is then sprayed into the blood rich, thin skinned area under the tongue and is absorbed into the bloodstream successfully. Sprays made in a facility that is FDA compliant, performs quality control on raw ingredients and practices GMP standards, will be more reliable than lesser quality products. Because high quality ingredients and proper homeopathic manufacturing are not inexpensive, low-priced products cannot contain the high quality ingredients, nor contain the required proper homeopathic manufacturing that ensures optimum effectiveness.

Homeopathic forms are safer. GH injections can flood the body with too much HGH that may cause the pituitary gland to stop secreting natural growth hormone. GH has a life of 90 minutes in the body before it is destroyed. Therefore, if you inject GH once a day in large dose, after an hour and a half the body will discard what's left. The results are lost GH because of the lack of the body's ability to absorb this much at one time. This would be similar to eating 500 grams of protein at one meal for the whole entire day. The body couldn't absorb it and it would make you sick, forcing your body to discard it. The same applies for GH. Taking homeopathic GH is efficient because these small doses when administered frequently allow your pituitary gland to increase production naturally which allows you near complete absorption.

Research shows that positive changes usually take place in one to six months or more with using Homeopathic HGH. Your Growth Hormone levels may have been extremely low and it will take time to elevate them to desired levels. If you smoke, drink, have a poor diet or don't exercise, it may take longer. At times the body can shift into neutral and some results seem to diminish. Reasons for this could be nothing more than the body resting or using the GH to rebuild tissue. *Be patient and levels should return.*

According to Dr. Rosen, M.D. and Dr. G.Johannsson, M.D. from the University Hospital in Goteborg, Sweden, "Years of research have shown that homeopathic remedies work the same as their material counterparts but without the side effects. Homeopathics are gentle, safe and very effective. The homeopathic form of GH does not interfere with any other remedy, supplement or medicine that an individual might take."[4]

Using the homeopathic form of GH does not seem to interfere with any other remedy, supplement, or medicine that an individual might take. Other reasons to select the homeopathic form over injections is that homeopathic GH is easier to obtain and use than injections, is less expensive and from *The Journal of the American Medical Association,* September 2, 1998 "In clinical practice, homeopathics have demonstrated effectiveness repeatedly, bringing the body closer to homeostasis [internal balance]."

How Homeopathic HGH works

The pituitary gland is a small peanut-shaped "master gland" located at the base of the brain. The pituitary gland not only controls physical growth, but also regulates other glands throughout the body that produce hormones such as testosterone and estrogen. This gland naturally excretes GH at certain times, especially during the first 90 minutes of sleep. If you are supplementing with homeopathic HGH the body times the release of GH as opposed to injections which must be specific in their dosing times. Following the release of a burst of GH from the pituitary gland at night or during a between-meal period, the hormone is rapidly taken up by the liver which if thus informed chemically to make a myriad of growth factors. These are chemical messengers that instruct the various cells of the body, be they nerve, bone, skin, or muscle, to rebuild and repair themselves to their unique specifications. If the growth factors are lowered, less building occurs.

The homeopathic theory of dilution and succussion shows that these smaller molecules can penetrate the cells more easily. A homeopathic oral spray is absorbed into the cells of the mucous membrane, going directly to the pituitary gland and avoiding possible interaction in the process of being digested. The factor that is measured in the blood to determine an average person's daily GH secretion is called IGF-1. It is this lab test for IGF-1 that measures the result of your GH secretion. It is not advised for people under 30 to take HGH as their long bone growth is still undergoing changes.

The technical explanation: GHRH (Growth Hormone releasing hormone) is released from neurosecretory nerve terminals of arcuate neurons, and is carried by the hypothalamo-hypophyseal portal system to the anterior pituitary gland where it stimulates growth hormone (GH) secretion by stimulating the GHRH receptor. The GHRH in turn motivates the anterior lobe of the pituitary to release Growth Hormone. Somatostatin (growth-hormone-inhibiting hormone) is used by the hypothalamus to stop GH production when needed. GH then travels to the liver and causes growth factors- IGF-I and IGF-II (insulin-like growth factor I and II) to be released.

Results time line (average)

After first month or two:
• Decrease in weight
• Increase in sexual desire.
• Improved stamina.
• Better & sounder sleep, feeling more refreshed upon awakening. Increase in energy.
• More optimistic attitude and better sense of humor.

After third or fourth month.
• Improved muscle tone.
• Improvement in nail growth.
• Better digestion.
• Weight loss.
• Enhanced sexual function.
• Improvement to skin tone.
• Increase in strength.

Fifth Month and Beyond
• Muscle size increases, especially if exercising.
• Less pain.
• Improved nail growth (sign of protein, nutrient assimilation).
• Impressive weight loss and reduction of inches, since fat is reduced and muscle tissue is increased and toned.
• Thickening of skin and greater elasticity.
• Thickening of hair with a shiny and healthy appearance.
• Improvement to skin texture and appearance (including skin discoloration

*Please note that everyone is different – some may notice immediate, dramatic results, while others experience more subtle benefits. Consider the condition you are now in and how long you have been in this condition. Even if you do not notice immediate results, the GH is probably still working.

➢ Shake the bottle of HGH spray before using. There's no need to take food with this supplement--in fact, if you take it after eating, wait at least 30 minutes past the meal before using the spray. Likewise, allow at least 30 minutes after using the spray before you eat. According to homeopathic principles, it is recommended that food, toothpaste, chewing gum, coffee, mint, etc. be avoided for a half-hour before and after taking GH so there will be less likelihood of interference with the homeopathic action.

➢ Spray under your tongue two or three times in the morning, in the late afternoon and at bedtime--check your product literature for the exact dosage. We advise that you take HGH five days a week, then skip two days, so the body's receptor sites can "rest" and let the body use the hormone and create its own.

➢ Hold the liquid HGH spray under your tongue for at least 20 seconds without swallowing. Once the 20 seconds have passed, you can go ahead and swallow.

If you are sensitive to alcohol (which is often used in homeopathic products) the drops can be placed in a small amount (3 ounces) of warm, not hot water for one minute to evaporate the alcohol. You may also apply the HGH Topically to the underside of the wrists, stomach or inside of the thigh as an alternative, but if possible take HGH orally. Keep HGH, and all supplements, away from extreme heat or light and away from drugs, toxic substances, x-ray, and EMFs (electro-magnetic fields).

During the healing process, some people may feel symptoms such as a stronger heartbeat, headache, upset stomach, etc. To diffuse these symptoms you can temporarily cease to take the GH or reduce the amount of GH or change the doses to once a day or once every other day. People may experience a slight recurrence of aches and pains in areas from locations of past old injuries. Homeopathic principles claim that this is part of a healing "crisis" in areas where energy was previously blocked. This is called "retracing" or "aggravation." To mitigate this reduce your dosage of GH while the body gets used to the therapy and reintroduce more gradually.

Be patient. Listen to your body. Start HGH therapy slowly and increase dosage and frequency with which you take it over time. Give the body time to react. If you are a diabetic or have any medical condition, consult your doctor or holistic physician before taking HGH or any supplement. Research has revealed that some diabetics on HGH therapy decreased their need for insulin.

And be advised that product label information is for educational and informational purposes only. Always consult a health professional should the need arise.

Chapter Four

Testing with Homeopathic HGH

A total of 162 healthy people, ages 18-72 years old, were evaluated for serum IGF-1 levels in three differently designed phase I/II, double-blind placebo-controlled trials (DBPCT). The Seattle Study, was a 30-day study on 15 subjects, 18-57 years old, who exercised 3 to 5 times per week. The Santa Fe, Proving Study, included 46 subjects, 19-59 years old, who participated in a homeopathic proving in which the identity of the test substance was not revealed. The Boulder Study, enrolled 101 individuals who did not exercise regularly, 29-72 years old, in a 42-day, DBPCT with a crossover after 21 days to the opposite test substance, i.e., treatment was crossed to placebo and vice versa.

There were three major findings from these different double-blind placebo-controlled studies. The first finding was that oral administration of HhGH produced physiologic effects. Rises in serum IGF-1 levels occurred with both 6C + 100C + 200C HhGH and 6X + 12C HhGH compared to transient rises and final downward trends in subjects who were on placebo. It is important to note that 6X + 12C HhGH stimulated a rapid 18 ± 10 percent physiologic rise in serum IGF-1 level after only 7 days in Santa Fe subjects who were not aware of what substance was being tested. Although homeopathy's molecular mechanism of action remains to be fully elucidated, HhGH clearly evokes quantifiable physiologic changes in the bloodstream.

The next finding showed that similar to injectable HGH, chewable tablets of Homeopathic HGH had positive effects on lean body mass, produced weight and fat loss, relieved fatigue, produced body shape changes, and improved psychologic well-being. The homeopathic HGH also improved self-perceived measures related to quality of life significantly, such as energy increase, weight loss, improved vision, increased libido, improved sleep quality, improved breathing, and improved skin softness. Thus, an oral formulation that was at least 4000 times lower in concentration than an injectable HGH provided some of the same benefits of the injectable HGH without its side effects.

Oral administration of HhGH lowered systolic blood pressure after 3 and 6 weeks, depending upon the formula that was used. Injectable hGH at 700 μg per day, 3 times per week, for 6 months, corrected systolic heart function that was caused by left-ventricle low-mass index. The degree of change in systolic function induced by HhGH requires further and more extensive clinical study. Subjects who enrolled in this study reported unique self-perceived benefits, far above the placebo effect and never-before associated with hGH injections. For example, subjects reported relief from bleeding gums, less phlegm build-up, relief from coughing, relief from anger, relief from apathy, and relief from urogenital discharges. These unique characteristics derived from HhGH underlie the possibility that a different signaling pathway is utilized than the pathway commonly outlined by molecular biologists.

Another significant implication of these findings relates to the other part of Hahnemann's Law of Similars, which states: "Whatever symptoms and syndromes a substance causes in large or toxic doses, it can heal when given in specifically prepared, exceedingly small homeopathic doses." Forty-nine subjects who received HhGH in these three differently designed studies reported relief from symptoms that they reported when they entered the studies. Symptoms relieved by HhGH treatment often matched the symptoms known to be caused by toxic doses of injectable hGH. Specifically relieved above placebo were headaches, edema, pain, and anxiety. Reductions in systolic blood pressure from HhGH are consistent with the findings that excessive hGH in patients with acromegaly correlated directly with cardiac abnormalities.[5]

A study done by Dr. Sydney Saffron was devised to test the clinical response to the homeopathic HGH formulation, as well as measure the changes in Free IGF-1 in saliva, to determine if measurable changes in body chemistry were occurring as predicted, and if the patient's symptoms correlated. The double-blind study included both men and women in several age brackets ranging from 25 -50 and 50+. The symptoms to be rated included: vision, skin condition, energy level, blood pressure, muscle strength, mental clarity, memory retention, joint movement, sleeping pattern, and overall health. All patients (who were required to be non-smokers) did a saliva sample at the beginning and end of the one month to measure for IGF-1, which is increased by growth hormone. Therapeutic, pharmaceutical doses have been shown to increase the levels. It was not clear how much impact there would be with homeopathic doses.

This was a small preliminary double-blind study meant to determine if homeopathic human growth hormone can show any objective changes in measurement of Salivary IGF-1 or any clinical symptom changes over a one month period of time in a group of patient volunteers of both sexes over age 25. Both of the study measurements definitely show an effect of this homeopathic formulation over a short period of time. The significant rise in measurable IGF-1 on the Saliva of 2.4 times the placebo effect is definitely dramatic, especially with a treatment that requires considerable compliance. The symptoms that showed significant improvement in average ratings between placebo and human growth hormone treatment groups included: vision (+11.16), skin condition(+11.03), energy levels(+11.03), overall health(+10.0), muscle strength(+8.97), joint movement(+6.1), and memory retention(+4.42).

Other studies show that GH can restore the body's ability to hydrate itself by retaining water in its tissues in a balanced form. We lose between 30-50 percent of our skin's water retention ability as we age. Properly dosed GH could bring an individual's hydration back to around 60 to 70 percent, that of a 20 or 30 year-old, making skin soft and reducing wrinkles. Researchers Trevor Cook, Ph.D, Dr. Emilio de Guidici, and Dr. Wolfgang Ludwig, a German biophysicist concluded that water molecules have a stable, hexagonal, lattice system, like an invisible honeycomb. This "honeycomb" can hold homeopathic "energies" and can change the structural shape of the water molecule lattice pattern! Succussing, or shaking, the homeopathic product seems to "transfer" the properties of the raw material to the water structure.

CHAPTER FIVE

HGH ENHANCERS

Specific ingredients can be added to a homeopathic HGH formula to increase its efficacy.

Avenia Sativa (Oats, Oat Straw):

This wonderful herb is thought to be soothing to the brain and nervous system, whilst at the same time increasing sexual desire, and performance. Avena sativa contains compounds which are both sedative and soothing to the brain and nervous system, hence it is said to be a good herb as a nerve restorative.[6] It is also shown to be helpful for digestion and depression, Herpes, arthritis, wrinkles, respiratory and immune support, anxiety disorders and A.D.D., migraine headaches, nicotine cravings and elevated cholesterol. Avena Sativa has the ability to increase testosterone levels by enhancing LH (luteinizing hormone) release. It has the effect of increasing free testosterone levels (the testosterone that can be used by the body). Research has been done that suggests Avena Sativa works by freeing up testosterone that is "stuck" to other compounds in the body. During the aging process, more testosterone gets bound, making it much less effective than free testosterone. Since Avena Sativa frees up this bound hormone, it makes it more efficient in the body.[7]

Glycyrrhiza glabra (European licorice):

Studies have shown that glycyrrhizin stimulates the excretion of hormones by the adrenal cortex. Glycyrrhizin has also shown estrogenic activity in laboratory animals, and is experimentally anti-inflammatory, anti-rheumatic, and antibacterial. Scientists have shown that licorice has an effect on the adrenals, helping to stimulate glucocorticoid production.[8] Glycyrrhiza is widely used in bronchial problems such as catarrh, bronchitis, cold, flu and coughs. It reduces irritation of the throat and yet has an expectorant action. It produces its demulcent and expectorant effects. It is used in relieving stress. It is a potent healing agent for tuberculosis, where its effects have been compared to hydrocortisone. Glycyrrhiza is also effective in helping to reduce fevers (glycyrretinic acid has an effect like aspirin), and it may have an antibacterial action as well. It is used in the treatment of chronic inflammations such as arthritis and rheumatic diseases, for chronic skin conditions, and autoimmune diseases in general.[9]

Amino Acids: Amino acids are reported to be an excellent way to enhance GH in the body especially when taken in the homeopathic (liquid) form.

•**L-arginine** – It is necessary for the production of protein. L-arginine also helps rid the body of ammonia (a waste product) and stimulates the release of insulin, and boosts immunity and healing. Arginine plays an important role in cell division and the healing of wounds, quickens repair time of damaged tissue, helps decrease blood pressure in clinical hypertensive subjects and enhances the release of hormones. In addition, L-arginine is used to make nitric oxide (a compound that relaxes the blood vessels).[10]

•**L-Glutamine** – L-glutamine supplements are often used to increase muscle mass, facilitate protein synthesis and cellular energy. L-glutamine is also essential to proper function of the immune system. In addition, L-glutamine appears to play a role in brain function and digestion. L-glutamine has been studied extensively over the past 10–15 years and has been shown to be useful in treatment of injuries, trauma, burns, and treatment-related side-effects of cancer as well as in wound healing for postoperative patients. Glutamine is also marketed as a supplement used for muscle growth in weightlifting, bodybuilding, endurance, and other sports.[11]

•**Isoleucine** – It is an essential amino acid, which means that humans cannot synthesize it, so it must be ingested. It is know to increase endurance and help heal and repair muscle tissue and encourage clotting at the site of injury. This amino acid is especially important to serious athletes and body builders because its primary function in the body is to boost energy and help the body recover from strenuous physical activity.[12]

•**Lysine** – L-Lysine is a necessary building block for all protein in the body. L-Lysine plays a major role in calcium absorption; building muscle protein, recovering from surgery or sports injuries, and the body's production of hormones, enzymes, and antibodies. Lysine is important for proper growth, and it plays an essential role in the production of carnitine, a nutrient responsible for converting fatty acids into energy and helping to lower cholesterol. Lysine plays an important role in the formation of collagen, a substance important for bones and connective tissues including skin, tendon, and cartilage.[13]

•**Ornithine** –Ornithine may promote muscle-building activity in the body by increasing levels of growth-promoting (anabolic) hormones such as insulin and growth hormone. L-ornithine has an anti-fatigue effect in increasing the efficiency of energy consumption and promoting the excretion of ammonia. It is used to reduce stress and is frequently used by body-builders and weightlifters to increase levels of HGH.[14]

•**Valine** – It an essential amino acid needed for optimal growth in infants and for nitrogen equilibrium in adults. Valine has a stimulating effect and is needed for muscle metabolism, repair and growth of tissue and maintaining the nitrogen balance in the body.[15] Since it is a branched-chain amino acid, it can be used as an energy source in the muscles, and in doing so preserves the use of glucose.

Adjunct Immune Enhancers. In addition to your HGH protocol you may want to consider other supplements to boost your immune system. Recommendations include B-complex; vitamins A, C, E; and a good electrolyte-forming trace mineral concentrate. Greens such as spirulina, chlorophyll, kelp and chlorella are beneficial.

*Note: Some people use molecular releasers, enhancers or secretagogues to promote GH effectiveness. But when you use a non-homeopathic molecular enhancer or a releaser, you interrupt the body's natural feedback mechanism and speed up the receptor sites that are ready to bind to the GH. The receptor sites remain in a state of high stimulation and do not have time to rest. For that reason, some authorities advocate "cycling" molecular GH releasers, or taking them for briefer periods, with set intervals of rest. The same applies to the injectable GH.

Chapter Six
A Healthy Lifestyle and HGH Therapy

When we take Homeopathic HGH we do so for a reason and expect specific results. Not everyone will get all of these benefits from taking HGH. Remember, people are different and each individual has specific deficiencies and needs. Therefore, each of us may see different results. If you have a poor diet and live an unhealthy lifestyle the results you want may not materialize as quickly.

The first step to creating a healthier lifestyle is to watch your diet. From years of chemical pollution from environmental and dietary sources, our bodies may be fatigued from dealing with all these intruders. The accumulation of acidity (acid) in the blood and the cells is one of the principle causes of disease and death. Leading researchers have found that there is no natural death. All deaths from so-called natural causes are merely the end points of a progressive acid saturation (toxemia).

Nearly all cooked, fried and baked foods are acid forming. Almost all drugs, pills, patent medicines, drinks, tonics, wine, liquors, coffee, tea, chocolate, cocoa, and all manufactured foods are acid forming. All canned fruits almost without exception, are acid forming. Even if canned fruits and many other canned foods are not originally acid forming, they are made acid forming by processing; i.e. peeling, paring, cooking, sweetening, preserving, or by altering and disorganizing the food and fruit molecules by as microwave cooking and steaming thus destroying the vitamins of life.

Acid is one of the causes of gastritis, heartburn, burning in the chest, bloating, dullness, poor memory and low energy. Acidity also causes arthritis, urinary ailments, heart valve problems, and kidney problems. So long as we can keep the tissues nourished and secretions, stomach, blood and bones alkaline, we are healthy, youthful, vigorous, efficient, lively and strong.

It is improbable to get sick so long as the human body is alkaline. It is equally improbable to keep well when the system is in an acid condition. Human acidity leads to disease, operations, and an early funeral. An alkaline diet results in health, longevity, youth and beauty.

pH Balance and Electrolytes

Our body is always trying to maintain a proper acid/alkaline balance, called the pH balance. Again, when we are acidic from too many acid-forming foods, aging and many diseases, including cancer can occur. Our cellular metabolism becomes unhealthy and we soon start to feel the effects. If you want to determine whether you are acid or alkaline, it's easy. Purchase a roll of pH-testing paper and place in the urine stream taken when you first get up in the morning. Match the color with the color code on the pH paper box. Darker (numbers towards 8.0) is more alkaline, lighter (numbers toward 5.5) more acid. An optimum number is 6.4. You can also use your saliva first thing in the morning. The optimum number is 6.8.

To correct your pH it is necessary to avoid the foods we have just mentioned. And it is important to drink water with a higher pH. Distilled or Reverse Osmosis water is extremely pure, but since most of the minerals have been removed through the purification process, the pH is low. Even filtered tap water may not have adequate pH as the minerals may have been filtered out by the city water system. In order to bring that pH up you need to "spike" it with a good liquid electrolyte-forming trace-mineral supplement before you drink it. Since we are supposed to drink eight glasses of water each day, it's important to make sure it's pH balanced. In addition adding electrolytes to the water tends to energize the body's electrical system which depends on minerals for message transmission (neurotransmitter function).

Electrolytes are the basis of good health because they are used in the maintenance and repair of all tissues, the utilization of amino acid (cells and tissue 'building blocks'), and as the basis of every physical and neurological function. They maintain osmotic equilibrium of our cell walls and the internal water balance that enables muscles and nerves to contract and expand, and wounds to heal. They are also essential for growth and development of the bones as well as the organs.

Additionally, the electrolyte solution is responsible for carrying minerals and amino acids to all points of the body. HGH therapy that is used in conjunction with a good electrolyte solution can have more distinctive results. The proper amount of electrolytic minerals should be available from a healthy diet and water. But, because of the erosion of the earth's topsoil and lack of farmers remineralizing their soil, plants are lacking the minerals we need. This has rendered this mineral source grossly inadequate and your diet should be supplemented.

Exercise and HGH

In addition to avoiding junk foods and eating more vegetables (organic we hope), we recommend making sure you do not have a sedentary lifestyle. Many of our jobs require sitting for long periods of time and unless you go to a gym or get some form of exercise after work, we find that our body starts crying out for oxygen. Exercise sends a wake-up call to your pituitary. Just getting started in a weight lifting or running program will stimulate your pituitary gland to secrete higher growth hormone levels. I'm sure it is no surprise that getting oxygen into the cells, toning muscle, supporting your heart and lungs and creating endurance and stamina are benefits of exercise that you have heard many times before. But, what you may not know is how beneficial HGH is to your exercise program.

Imagine the accelerated influence of combining proper diet, exercise and HGH therapy. Older people may have limited strength and stamina that affects their ability to exert themselves to the point of making significant gains against heart disease and osteoporosis. Restoring growth hormone levels often increases their energy, strength and stamina so they are able to do exercises that previously seemed impossible.

We have observed wonderful results that homeopathic growth hormone has on increasing exercise potential. A 72-year old woman with chronic arthritis and stiffness, who had not been able to exercise, saw terrific results. After only one week on HGH she had more flexibility and reduced pain. This allowed her to walk everyday and increase her tolerance for weight-bearing exercise.

Many athletes use homeopathic HGH to enhance their training programs. HGH is involved in many physiological processes throughout life, including the turnover of muscle, bone and collagen, the regulation of fat metabolism and the maintenance of a healthier body composition in later life. The best exercise for sending GH levels surfing is weight resistance training. In combination with homeopathic HGH, lifting weights can do things to your body that you never dreamed possible. To the extent that gym workouts are more productive using homeopathic HGH oral spray, muscle gains will be generated. This is normal and natural.[16]

HGH works with exercise because when your body's levels of HGH are restored it has the ability to create new muscle cells and fibers, thus increasing muscle mass and definition. Due to the increased amount of lean muscle mass in the body as a result of a natural HGH releaser, the body is able to burn more fat as it works. Natural HGH also increases the amount of IGF-1 that is excreted by the liver. IGF-1 blocks the transportation of glucose into the cells. Because glucose isn't available for the cells to use as energy, the body is forced to burn fat instead, thus promoting a leaner and more toned figure. In addition HGH can increase your energy levels so exercising becomes fun and not a chore.

For those who are serious about building muscle, research shows that the best way to train for maximal HGH release is to keep your rest periods between sets to a minute or less and use moderately heavy weights, performing no more than 9-12 reps per set. The burning feeling you get while lifting weights after an intense set signals the brain to release growth hormone. Even so, the release is affected by the necessity of maintaining high intensity by using moderately heavy weights. This means that doing high-rep sets with light weights may cause a burning sensation in muscles, but won't promote HGH release.[17]

Sleep and HGH

We all need restful sleep, but statistics from the National Institute of Neurological Disorders and Stroke estimate that about 40 million people in the United States have chronic long-term sleep disorders and another 20 million people have problems sleeping. Recent studies have shown that human growth hormone could be used to treat sleep problems in older adults.

Sleep patterns change as we age, and older people exhibit different patterns of sleep than younger people. Older people are less efficient sleepers, taking longer to fall asleep and then stay in bed longer to get the same amount of sleep they got when the were younger. Older people tend to wake more easily and more often than younger people and report feelings of insomnia more often. Daytime sleep also leads to difficulty sleeping through the night.

An article published in the August 16, 2000 Journal of the American Medical Association reported a link between sleep disorders and a lack of natural HGH in the blood of 149 men aged between 16 and 83. The research is credited to a team led by Professor Eve van Cauter of the University of Chicago. HGH is produced naturally at night during deep sleep and was highest for the younger test subjects. Subjects aged 45 and older lost the ability to fall back in deep sleep when awakened during the night. In subjects over 50, sleep declined 27 percent per decade of age, and growth hormone secretion had decreased by 75. While the University of Chicago study did not link sleep reduction directly to a lack of human growth hormone, the research did show a link: Less HGH was produced by the body because of less deep sleep time. Other studies on HGH replacement therapy have confirmed patients taking synthetic HGH sleep better at night.[18]

Sexual Performance and HGH

Dr. Michael Klentze, Medical Director of the Klentze Institute of Anti-Aging in Munich, Germany, has reported that there is a direct correlation between diminished levels of HGH and sexual dysfunction.[19] The decline in a broad spectrum of hormones, including estrogen and testosterone, affects both our vitality and our desire for sex.

At puberty, when GH is at its peak, a boy is in almost a constant state of arousal. This lessens as he ages and by age 60 his interest in sex diminishes and his rate of impotence increases. Every study of male sexual function shows a decline with age. Clinical studies have shown that men who are experiencing varying degrees of erectile dysfunction have shown dramatic improvement from human growth hormone therapy.[20]

According to the classic survey by Kinsey, under the age of forty about two percent of men are impotent. By age eighty, 75 percent are incapable of having sex. In the first clinical analysis of the effects of GH replacement by Dr. Terry and Dr. Chein,[21] three-quarters of the 172 men tested said that they had an increase in sexual potency or frequency and 62 percent reported that they were able to maintain an erection for a longer period of time. A study by the Nottingham Health Profile reported that in a group of 302 elderly men who were taking HGH therapy, 75 percent reported an improvement in sexual potency while 62 percent had longer lasting erections.

Women don't have as much trouble reaching orgasm in their older years, but the loss of estrogen at menopause causes vaginal dryness and atrophy of the vaginal tissues. This can cause discomfort and lead many women to avoid intercourse. Their hormonal change can also reduce their libido, a factor in part attributed to lower levels of growth hormone. Women who add homeopathic HGH to their lifestyle regime have reported increased libido, heightened pleasure and the equivalent of greater potency in men in the form of multiple orgasms. It also has helped reduce post-menopausal symptoms. A fifty-four-year old patient had her hot flashes completely disappear with HGH. Her follicle-stimulating hormone levels (high FSH levels are an indication of subfertility and/or infertility) also dropped from 60 to 8, a normal level for pre-menopausal younger women.

How we think and feel about ourselves influences sexual functioning in both men and women. HGH has a direct effect on the biochemistry of the brain, which in turn controls cognition, emotion and mood. It also raises cellular metabolism and energy levels. The neurotransmitters, which are the chemical messengers in the brain, have receptors all over the body Sexual responsiveness is to a large degree determined by what happens with these neurotransmitters. When we feel good about ourselves we become more open to the sensual world around us and the feelings of touch and desire.

Select homeopathic formulas should contain a powerful and proprietary blend of natural ingredients designed to safely strengthen and empower the body's pituitary gland to operate at more youthful levels. A stronger and more youthful functioning pituitary gland may offer increased levels of HGH into the body's bloodstream.

Anti-Aging and HGH

Average life span and life expectancy in the United States have grown dramatically in this century, from about 47 years in 1900 to about 81 years in 2010. It is understood in many circles that we age because our hormone levels drop. Maintaining hormone levels can prevent age-related diseases and turn back our biological age, thereby increasing our health span and life expectancy. But above all it can improve our quality of life by bringing our hormone levels back to what they were when we were younger. Depending on the type of cell, these T cells reproduce every several months or years. You would think our young cells would prevent aging, but in fact a wrinkled mother skin cell will produce a wrinkled daughter skin cell and the body's cells know how old we are. This is because the information about our biological age is transmitted to the DNA by hormones. As hormone levels in the body decrease, less of the hormone is attached to the cell wall, and a weaker electrical signal is given to the DNA of the reproducing mother cell. This is the signal that tells the DNA that our body has aged, causing the daughter cells to be reproduced in the old or diseased state of the mother cells.

A solution to staving off this process is to increase the hormone levels, signaling the DNA of the mother cell to work again. Once the DNA receives the signal that the body is that of a 20-year-old, it will reproduce young, healthy daughter cells, and these cells will reverse our biological age.[22] Produced by glands, organs, and tissues, hormones are the body's chemical messengers, flowing through the blood stream and searching out cells fitted with special receptors. The female hormone, estrogen is produced mainly by the ovaries. It slows the bone thinning that accompanies aging and may help prevent frailty and disability. After menopause, fat tissue is the major source of a weaker form of estrogen than that produced by the ovaries. Melatonin hormone comes from the pineal gland. As it declines during aging, it may trigger changes throughout the endocrine system. The male hormone, testosterone is produced in the testes and may decline with age, though less frequently or significantly than estrogen in women. Researchers are investigating its ability to strengthen muscles and prevent frailty and disability in older men when administered as testosterone therapy for dehydroepiandrosterone, DHEA is produced in the adrenal glands. It is a weak male hormone and a precursor to some other hormones, including testosterone and estrogen. DHEA is being studied for its possible effects on selected aspects of aging, including immune system decline, and its potential to prevent certain chronic diseases, like cancer and multiple sclerosis.

In our estimation the brains behind hormone balancing is growth hormone. As we've mentioned before, this product of the pituitary gland appears to play a role in body composition and muscle and bone strength. It is released through the action of another trophic factor called growth hormone releasing hormone, which is produced in the brain. It works by stimulating the production of insulin-like growth factor, which comes mainly from the liver. Produced primarily in the liver, IGF-1 enters and flows through the blood stream, seeking out special IGF-1 receptors on the surface of various cells, including muscle cells Through these receptors it signals the muscle cells to increase in size and number, perhaps by stimulating their genes to produce more of special, muscle-specific proteins. Also involved at some point in this process are one or more of the six known proteins that bind with IGF-1; their regulatory roles are still a mystery.[23]

The action of growth hormone also may be intertwined with a cluster of other factors. Exercise stimulates a certain amount of GH secretion on its own, and obesity, depresses production of GH. Even the way fat is distributed in the body may make a difference; lower levels of GH have been linked to excess abdominal fat but not to lower body fat. HGH does not affect the root cause of aging, as measured by maximum lifespan, but it can certainly affect many of the manifestations of aging.[24]

You can use HGH as an anti-aging substance and in most cases you may notice that your skin is going to look ten years younger. If that is what you want, then you can start around the age of 50, depending on genetics and how many wrinkles you have at the onset. If you are into fitness and bodybuilding there is no better and faster solution than the HGH.

Chapter Seven

Testimonials*

Information on product used in these testimonials can be found in our chapter: Resource Directory

"I am 73 years-old and have always been active in sports. For over a year I had been having terrible pains in both hips from just walking. A couple of years earlier I had surgery for a torn rotator cuff. After a week and a half of taking Americare Homeopathic Oral Spray, all of a sudden I realized I had walked a mile with no pain at all. I also realized that my shoulder was no longer hurting. It was a miracle. I thought I was going to need hip replacements and I was dreading another shoulder surgery." -*Mr. J. Singer - Woodland Park, NJ*

"Ever since I have been taking Homeopathic Oral Spray, I have been able to double the energy I put into my workouts and I have lost weight. So my cardiologist said I can now reduce my daily heart medicine dosage. First time in 25 years! I am a firm believer in homeopathic HGH and will never stop taking the products!" -*Ms. M. Steele - Woodland Hills, CA*

"I have used three bottles of Homeopathic Oral Spray and my doctor asked me what I was doing differently. He said he noticed a change in me and it wasn't just the 52 pounds I had lost. I told him about the HGH product from Americare that I was taking and he wanted to know more about the product. I feel better physically - all over. Thank you for this product. I am even going to start my precious mother on it!" -*Ms. A. Graham - Kingsport, TN*

"I have been using homeopathic HGH drops for a short time now, and I am astonished and pleased about the results. On March 17th I fell and broke a rib and was also experiencing low back pain. Up to that time, I was exercising regularly. My ribs feel healed and now I have returned to exercising after only six weeks. I never dreamed this product could have this effect!" -*Ms. L. St. Paul, New Orleans, LA*

"I have been using Homeopathic HGH Therapy spray on a regular basis for about eight months now. I can tell a great deal of my energy has been regained. I am 62 years-old and have been active all my life. I was starting to slow down and was losing my enthusiasm for life. Now I am back on track, watching my weight and getting daily exercise. I thank you for introducing me to this wonderful formula!" -*Ms L. Kappes, Soquel, CA.*

"I know that without HGH I would have been dead at least two years ago. I was at death's door when I began taking this miracle in a bottle two years ago and was hard pressed for actually taking it. But, I believe that it saved me, if only for awhile. I want you to know that I truly believe in this product and I believe it has kept me here for two years. Las Vegas is known for gambling and I gambled on this product and won the golden card and most significant prize. Thank you from the bottom of my heart." – *Carol B., Crevve Ct, IL*

"When I was twenty, thirty and I think forty years-old I slept like a baby. I used to feel sorry for friends that had insomnia because it sounded so awful. But now I'm 54 and I'm not sure when my sleeping problems started, but they grew and grew. I couldn't go to sleep at night. I would read a book until I could hardly keep my eyes open but as soon as I turned the light off I'd be wide awake! Maybe, I would read for hours and then get up and eat a bowl of cereal. That might work, but I got fat in the stomach. Sometimes I would go to sleep alright, but wake up all through the night. I tried a lot of supplements because I like alternative and take zero prescriptions. But nothing worked. One day a lady called me on the phone and talked me into trying the homeopathic HGH spray. I was hesitant because it was not cheap! Now I've been taking it for several months and guess what? It is worth every penny and more because I sleep well every night now. I go to sleep quickly and sleep all night. Thank you, Thank you, Thank you."- *Pam S., Gainesville, FL*

"Thank you truly for the introduction to the homeopathic HGH. I have been successfully taking the time to use this product. It has given me such a new direction in my life. I strongly would like to tell all individuals to use this on a daily basis. Spray as often as you can and you will receive all the benefits of this great product. I have told several of my family members and friends how this new product formula truly works. Believe me I don't want to live without it. So, all clients and new clients will enjoy this product as much as possible. Keep on spraying as I do and you will always keep getting fantastic and wonderful results." –*Chaz S., Langhorn PA*

"I have been using the homeopathic HGH product for the past four years. All of my friends guess my age at around seventy. I also feel and act like a 70-year old being as active as I am. No one including myself can believe that my age is 90. Thanks for starting me on your product." –*Sid C, Indio CA*

"I started taking the product on January 10th, 2011. I have two heart stents in my arteries, I'm a controlled diabetic, have high blood pressure, cholesterol and triglycerides (now normal), skin problems (pre-cancerous). I've had laser surgery for glaucoma in both eyes, have chronic dry eyes, tinnitus in my ear, colon problems and sever constipation most of my life. I'm 70 years old and since starting the HGH I've lost 15 pounds, my double chin is going away. What to me looked like hog jaws, and my wrinkles in my face are tightening. I've had people come up and ask me what I'm doing. I tell them about homeopathic HGH and how to get it. Even my gray hair seems to be turning back to normal color. Also I have COPD and notice it's getting better. The ringing in my ears isn't as loud and the moisture in my eyes is improving. I can't wait to see what four more months will bring. God Bless the discovery and production of homeopathic HGH. I wish I'd discovered it twenty years ago." –*Saundra R., Ro Ann, IN*

"Let me identify myself. I am a 61 year-old female with Lupus, fibromyalgia, arthritis and spinal injury called Trans Verse Myalytis since 2003. I have right leg paralysis which causes me to be in a wheelchair. I received a call one day and was introduced to homeopathic HGH. I received my shipment in a few days. I take many medications (12) per day. After my first month of HGH I was down to 11 meds per day and my joint pain had decreased tremendously. I am now off the steroids completely. Each month my medication, pain and weight decreased. At the end of my three months on HGH I have lost 40 pounds and my meds are down to five per day. I would recommend this to anyone with autoimmume disorder." –Geraline D., San Antonio TX

"When I ordered my homeopathic HGH supplement, I was afraid to try it. Even my Doctor advised that I not use it. However, when I was told the product was homeopathic and would not cause any adverse reactions, I proceeded with my order. Now having used it, I must tell you I love it! After using it for about three weeks, one night I found myself in the kitchen – around 9 p.m. baking cookies. Normally when I arrive home from work, make dinner and do the dishes, I am so tired I do nothing else. I had such an abundance of energy, I could not sit still. The only thing to which I could attribute this burst of energy was the HGH supplement. Thanks for encouraging me to use it." – *Liz. E, Jackson MI*

CHAPTER EIGHT

QUESTIONS AND ANSWERS

Q: **What are the differences between injections versus capsules, powders and an oral spray?** HGH injections require a dosage of 4 to 8 IU's weekly and is administered twice daily by an anti-aging medical practitioner at a cost of $800 to $1,500.00 a month! Capsules and powders are taken orally into the digestive system and are broken down by stomach bile and acids. Powders have to be measured and mixed prior to assimilation. Homeopathic HGH Oral Spray is sprayed directly into the mouth three times a day and is absorbed directly into the mucus membrane. It is safe, efficient and cost effective.

Q: **How long before I see and feel results?** Some of the improvements reported have taken place over a period of 6 to 12 months. *results vary on individuals*

Q: **Does homeopathic spray have a shelf life and does it have to be kept in the refrigerator?** One manufacturer we spoke to, Americare, commented that their product has a shelf life of two years and because it is stabilized by a calcium carbonate and distilled water, there is no need to refrigerate. However, it is advised to keep your product out of extreme heat or direct sunlight.

Q: **How does HGH act in my body, and how is it measured?** Following the release of a burst of GH from the pituitary gland at night or during a between-meal period, the hormone is rapidly taken up by the liver which if thus informed chemically to make a myriad of growth factors. These are chemical messengers that instruct the various cells of the body, be the nerve, bone, skin, or muscle, to rebuild and repair themselves to their unique specifications. If the growth factors are lowered, less building occurs. The factor that is measured in the blood to determine an average person's daily GH secretion is called IGF-1. It is this lab test for IGF-1 that measures the result of your GH secretion.

Q: What age is best to take Americare Homeopathic Spray? And is it safe for children? The best age to take homeopathic HGH is when the individual starts taking an interest in keeping their youthful levels. This can be from the late twenties to thirties.

Q: What else can be done to restore my youthful levels of GH? If you wish to pursue greater HGH replacement, we recommend you consult a physician that has a background in anti-aging.

Q: What research and studies are available on Growth Hormone? Today there are over two hundred books on Anti-aging hormones and replacements on the market. Visit your nearest book store soon!

Q: What if I stop taking GH? Will I instantly "age"? Not right away. As the cells lose their "youth" memory you may see changes, but restarting HGH therapy should restore the benefits. Once a person has taken HGH and seen the results, s/he generally wants to continue taking it. There are supplements everyone should take throughout life for health maintenance. Homeopathic GH is affordable, so you don't have to worry about not being able to continue taking it.

Q: Is it possible to take too much *homeopathic* HGH? It is possible to take too much of anything, including food and water! Homeopathic GH is gentle and safe and since "too much" varies from person to person they may or may not experience temporary negative or uncomfortable symptoms. Reducing the amount of GH taken, or temporarily discontinuing the GH, easily alleviates these symptoms. When symptoms subside, the dosage can be gradually increased.

Q: Will HGH interfere with medications, herbs, etc.? The homeopathic form of HGH has not been reported to interfere with any medications or other substances, including supplements.

Q: Does HGH have side effects? Early side effects with injectable GH were mainly due to dosages that were too high and being taken at the wrong time. If you look at all the worldwide GH studies, we see that the few side effects that did occur resulted from too high a dose of injectable GH and from taking it either at the wrong time, or at incorrect intervals. Dr. Chein and Dr. Terry have found that they eliminated side effects by administering a low dose first thing in the morning and last thing in the evening. They followed this plan consistently, six days a week, and allowed one-day off so the receptor sites could relax and the body could create and process the GH. Some people may experience slight "detoxification" effects or temporary "tiredness". Therapeutic homeopathic agents encourage the body toward health without artificially suppressing symptoms. If you experience uncomfortable detoxifying, stop or reduce the frequency and dosage until the effects pass (two to three days or longer), and drink lots of electrolyte water. The body may experience a past health condition or an old injury. When this happens, the body is "cleansing" itself of that past condition. This is similar to detoxification.[25] Interestingly enough, the best results were obtained with the smallest dosages of GH. Without knowing it at the time, studies were pointing to the effectiveness of homeopathy!

Homeopathic HGH is the safest, most sophisticated and effective growth hormone delivery system ever seen. Combined with years of scientific research along with the benefits, safety and effectiveness of 200 years of use of homeopathy.

Q: Can GH cause cancer or speed up cancer or affect the heart or liver? Dr. Chein and Dr. Terry treated nearly 1,000 people who were at risk for cancer, and not one developed cancer! In fact, one man with prostate cancer actually had his cancer disappear with GH therapy. Dr. Ronald Klatz is one of the world's top experts on GH and President of the American Academy of Anti-Aging. He carefully studied this area and concluded that GH gives a "protective effect," because it "revives and rejuvenates the immune system." Some studies have shown that GH actually strengthens the heart. Others show that some damaged or diseased livers and other organs have been brought back to a state of health with GH therapy

Q: Will Homeopathic HGH cause tissue, bones and organs to grow abnormally large? No. Problems of this sort are linked to injectable molecular GH when used in too high a dosage over a prolonged period of time.

wo tests, as mentioned by Roy Walford M.D. in his book, *The 120 Year Diet: How to Double Your Vital Years* are mentioned here. These can give you an indication of how your skin is aging and how you measure up in reaction time.

1. Weight over the bar Skin Flexibility Test:
As you age, you lose elastin and collagen along with skin moisture, and the skin becomes less elastic. GH tones the skin, and a lack of GH could be one indicator of sagging, inflexible skin. To test your skin's resiliency, use your thumb and forefinger to pinch the skin on the back of your hand for 5 seconds
You must time how long it takes the skin to go back to its normal place. Here are rate times (note: time will vary):
a. Forty-five and fifty Years- 5 seconds
b. Sixty Years- 10-15 seconds
c. Seventy Years- 35-50 seconds

1. Ruler Test
This is to test reaction time. Take an eighteen-inch ruler (wooden) and get a partner to hold the ruler at the top with the eighteen-inch mark at the bottom with your fingers in between. Use your dominant thumb and middle finger which should be three and a half inches apart (equally on both sides of the ruler) at the eighteen inch point. Your partner is to drop the ruler without telling you and you try to catch the falling ruler. Do this procedure three times and get an average.
Illustration: Here are the averages for people in their twenties and sixties:
a. Twenty year-old - 11 inch marker
b. Sixty year old- 6 inch marker

End Notes

(Endnotes)

1 http://www.AACE.com and Ref. 14.

2 http://en.wikipedia.org/wiki/Growth_hormone

3 Kleijnen, J., Knipschild, P., ter Riet, G. Clinical trials of homeopathy. *Br Med J* 302:316-323, 1991.

4 http://www.hmedicine.com/homeopathy/information/hgh_anti-aging.php

5 http://research-data.com/Latest-Findings/HGH-Study.htm

6 http://www.herbwisdom.com/herb-avena-sativa.html

7 http://www.trulyhuge.com/avena-sativa-benefits.html

8 http://www.stevenfoster.com/education/monograph/licorice.html

9 http://glycyrrhiza-glabra.101herbs.com/

10 http://en.wikipedia.org/wiki/Arginine

11 http://altmedicine.about.com/od/herbsupplementguide/a/L-Glutamine.htm

12 http://www.vitaminstuff.com/amino-acid-isoleucine.html

13 http://www.umm.edu/altmed/articles/lysine-000312.htm#ixzz2AtXqidnj

14 Fogelholm et al. (1993) "Low-dose amino acid supplementation: no effects on serum human growth hormone and insulin in male weightlifters", International Journal of Sport Nutrition 3(3):290-7

15 http://medical-dictionary.thefreedictionary.com/valine

16 http://EzineArticles.com/4091378

17 http://www.fitflex.com/hghrelease.html

18 iHGH Growth Hormone for Sleep Disorder | eHow.com

19 http://EzineArticles.com/6943902

20 http://research-data.com/Latest-Findings/HGH-Study.htm

21 Dr. Ronald Klatz, *Grow Young with HGH*

22 Dr. Cass Terry, M.D., PhD, and Dr. Edmund Chein MD, Effects of Raising HGH levels on 202 patients (low dose)Medical College of Wisconsin

23 http://www.totalhormonegenetherapy.com/hgh_doctor.html

24 http://www.antiagingresearch.com/life_span.shtml

25 Davis, Howard, Dr. *Feeling Younger with Homeopathic HG*H, Safe Goods Publishing

Results from Boulder studies[26]

Symptom	Boulder 6X + 12C	Boulder 6C
Constitutional		
Relief from fatigue	70%	69%
Weight loss	66%	50%
Skin and extremities		
Relief from dry scaly skin	75%	58%
Greater softness/suppleness	25%	60%
Eyes		
Visual improvements	50%	82%
Relief from floaters	60%	44%
Oral		
Bleeding gums stopped	100%	50%
Respiratory		
Less coughing	56%	100%
Less shortness of breath	75%	100%
Less phlegm buildup	50%	71%
Gastrointestinal/abdominal		
Less pain	0%	83%
Less bloating	67%	80%
Less abdominal obesity	50%	73%
Urogenital		
Relief from discharges	100%	67%
Decreased libido *a*	100%	57%
Increased libido *a*	100%	60%
Musculoskeletal		
Improved physical appearance	**50%**	**80%**
relief from jaw pain	**100%**	**80%**
Psychologic		
Relief from apathy	**100%**	**80%**
Relief from anxiety	**83%**	**60%**
Relief from anger	-	**83%**
Improved quality of sleep	**57%**	**45%**
Neurologic		
Relief from headaches	**64%**	**69%**
Relief from weakness in arms and legs	**40%**	**100%**
Relief from joint swelling	**100%**	**100%**
Relief from knee swelling	**100%**	**100%**

Resources:

AMERICARE HOMEOPATHIC HGH SPRAY
This product is 100% Homeopathic and is all natural, no animal or human cadavers were used in its production. It is sprayed directly into the mouth three times a day and is absorbed directly into the mucus membrane. It is safe, efficient and cost effective. 191 Trace amino acids are in the product in addition to Avena Sativa, and Glycyrrhiza glabra. You can expect the finest, safest and most proven ingredients in our formulas. We use state-of-the-art nutraceutical manufacturing facilities that practice GMP Procedures (Good Manufacturing Practice) in the process of making their product, and sell to consumers that want effective, powerful products that work!!!! www.Americarenow.com   (800) 498-9799

BROAD-SPECTRUM TRACE MINERAL FORMULA
Electrolyte-forming trace minerals keep the signals from the brain to the rest of the body in motion. Since most water has been filtered, most of the trace minerals have been removed. Trace minerals create the electrolytic charge needed to support the brain. *electroBlast's* electrolyte-formula trace-mineral concentrate restores this deficiency. This product is easily squirted into water or any beverage. As compared to most electrolyte drinks electroBlast contains no artificial colors or flavors. It is just pure electrolytes in a convenient 2 oz. pump bottle. 888-217-7233 www.electroblast.com

HORMONE TESTING KITS
Aging can begin as a result of hormone imbalances that can also change sexual desire and performance. Simple saliva tests for determining hormone levels can be taken in your own home and sent to a professional lab for analysis. Results will be sent directly back to you. 888-217-7233
www.ForeverYoungCooperative.com/testing-kits.html

OTHER BOOKS FROM SAFE GOODS

- *The Secrets of Staying Young* $ 11.95
- *Worse Than Global Warming* $ 9.95
- *The Rivers Bend* $ 18.95
- *Letters from my Son* $ 22.95
- *QiGong Awakens* $ 12.95
- *Flying Above the Glass Ceiling* $ 14.95
- *No Scrip for my Journey* $ 29.95
- *Spirit and Creator* $ 29.95
- *2012 Airborne Prophesy* $ 16.95
- *What is Beta Glucan* $ 4.95
- *The Minerals you Need* $ 4.95
- *Eye Care Naturally* $ 8.95
- *Rx for Computer Eyes* $ 8.95
- *Wrinkles No More* $ 4.95
- *Zeolite* $ 4.95

For a complete listing of books visit our website:
safegoodspub.com

About the Author

Howard Peiper N.D, is a doctor
of naturopathic medicine. While
beginning his career in optometry,
he was immediately drawn to
the field of alternative health.
In 1972, he received his degree
in Naturopathy. After a decade
in private practice, Dr. Peiper
moved on to become a successful
writer, speaker, and consultant.
Over the years, his cutting-
edge articles have appeared in
numerous medical journals and
magazines. He also serves on
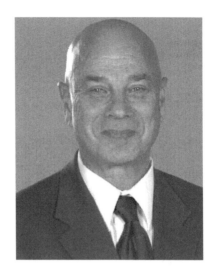
the medical advisory board for several nutritional companies. Dr.
Peiper has written several best-selling titles including *The ADD and
ADHD Diet* and *New Hope for Serious Disease.* He is a frequent
guest speaker on radio and television and has hosted his own radio
shows including the award-winning TV show, Partners in Healing.
Currently, Dr. Peiper lives in the Tampa Bay area and continues to
travel and lecture throughout the world.

Editor *Nina Anderson, C.NLP, SPN*
Nina Anderson is an ISSA certified Specialist in Performance
Nutrition, Neuro Linguistic Practitioner and author of 18 books on
natural health and aviation, including *The Secrets of Staying Young,
Analyzing Sports Drinks* and *Overcoming Senior Moments.*

NOTES

Notes

Notes

Notes

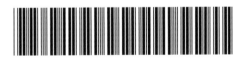